HOW TO MAINTAIN ANTI-AGING APPEARANCE

Mastering the Art of staying Young

Maya Glenn

1

INTRODUCTION

Aging is a fact of life; it's a process we can't escape. Until the day comes when scientists unlock a genetic miracle to halt aging, we all have to accept that our bodies will change as we grow older, year by year, even if blowing out a growing number of birthday candles is a tradition many of us abandon after childhood.

However, while getting older is a certainty, the manner in which we age is something we can influence. You have a voice in shaping your appearance, your health, and your overall well-being. Granted, some factors are left to chance, but a significant portion of your aging process is influenced by your diet, your daily habits, and your overall outlook on life.

In this program, we're going to dive into the strategies for maximizing your body's potential, enhancing your appearance, sharpening your mind, and even advancing your career, regardless of your age. This program is designed to reveal the keys to aging with elegance and vitality, whether you're male or female, and no matter the challenges you face.

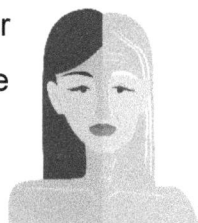

You'll come to understand that it's possible for your body to support you throughout your entire life journey – that dealing with persistent aches, pains, and skin issues isn't a foregone conclusion. We'll explore ways to ensure you keep flourishing right up until your final moments on this planet.

Do you need this Book?

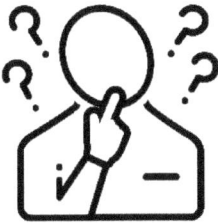

Let's get one thing straight before diving in: this program is meant for everyone, no matter the stage of life you're in. You might be entering your golden years, thinking it's too late to make a change because of the arthritis setting in or the wrinkles crinkling. But that's far from the truth! This guide is packed with methods and tips that can help turn back the clock on cell, brain, and joint damage—and you'll notice some pretty impressive results pretty quickly.

On the flip side, maybe you're on the younger side, feeling invincible, or haven't given a second thought to aging. Well, if you're past 25, it's time to wake up because your body is already on the downhill slide. Every day you shrug off this reality, you're basically fast-forwarding to an older, more worn-out version of yourself.

The key is to start taking care of your health now. The advice here isn't just for immediate gains; it's your shield against the visible signs of aging that could creep up on you in a year or less. It's about reaping the benefits today and safeguarding your future self.

For the young ones reading this, it all boils down to your vision for the future. Can you think ahead and plan for the long term, or are you stuck in the instant gratification of the present?

Before you decide whether this is worth your time, picture a day down the line—maybe a few years from now, maybe several decades. There's a good chance you'll get an invite to a school or college reunion. Imagine showing up and turning heads, looking absolutely fabulous. If you're single, you might just catch the eye of the best-looking people from your younger days. If you're taken, you can still strut your stuff and show off how amazing you've managed to look.

Or, you could ignore all the advice laid out in this program, live in the moment, and then show up to that reunion looking worn out and run down. You don't want to be the one people gossip about, saying, "Wow, they really didn't take care of themselves."

So, think about it. The choice is yours.

Chapter 1

The Influence of Personal Habits

Amazing celebs who've aged like fine wine.

You've probably noticed among your circle and even on TV how a person's lifestyle can really affect how they age. But it's more profound than you might think. These factors can create a significant impact that's more than just skin deep. Just look at some folks you know who are in their 40s, 50s, or 60s, and see the variety. Some 40-somethings could be mistaken for 30-year-olds, not just because of how they look, but also because of their zest for life, energy, and outlook.

Yet, there are others in their 40s who seem worn out and aged beyond their years. You know who I mean: they often have sun-damaged skin, large families, and a constant cigarette in hand. I want you to check out this guy called Aaron Marino, also known as 'Alpha'. He's got a YouTube channel about style and grooming, offering advice on skincare, seasonal fashion, and even tips on dating and making money.

Now, Aaron is 41, and he's killing it. He's practically wrinkle-free, has a killer body, dresses sharply, and exudes confidence. At 41, he's a prime example of how the right lifestyle choices can make a difference. And you can see similar effects in

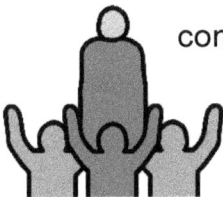

celebrities. Take Angelina Jolie, who at 42 looks amazing despite a tough life. She's got the resources, like a team of experts, to keep her looking great.

Consider Jennifer Lopez at 47 and Jennifer Aniston at 48 – they defy their age, and JLo's dancing background plays a part in her youthful appearance. Dancing is vital for staying young and healthy – just look at Bruce Forsyth dancing at 89!

Let's talk about some older stars. Arnold Schwarzenegger is still thriving at 69, having reclaimed his physique post-governorship. Sylvester Stallone, at 70, is still rocking Hollywood and has a sculpted body. Sure, they might have had a bit of help, but there are legal ways to tap into that same energy.

For female role models, look at Joanna Lumley at 71, still gorgeous and active in her career, or Helen Mirren, who at 71 continues to represent beauty and anti-aging brands.

So, it's not just men who can maintain their style into their 70s. Women are doing it with flair too!

Discover how to snag their age-defying tricks for yourself.

So, as we've discussed, maintaining a fabulous look and youthful energy is definitely achievable at virtually any stage in life. Of course, there's a bit of chance involved. For instance, if you have a hip injury that requires surgery, bouncing back from that can be tough. And if your genes make you more prone to conditions like Alzheimer's or arthritis, you're looking at a steeper climb.

But no matter what cards you're dealt, your lifestyle choices and self-care habits can have a transformative impact. Picture yourself two decades from now. Envision the best and worst versions of your future self. Which path will you choose?

We've seen plenty of celebrities who defy age with their stunning looks and vigor, but let's be real—they've got some advantages, like teams of beauty experts and access to the fanciest age-defying products money can buy. Chances are, you aren't swimming in that kind of luxury.

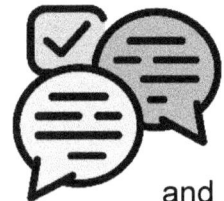

However, you can still adopt a similar mindset. It's all about investing in yourself and your future health and happiness. These stars understood that their appearance and energy were key to their success, refusing to let grey hair or a receding hairline dictate their careers.

You might not be in the spotlight, but investing in your future holds the same truth for you. Neglecting your well-being can impact your earnings, activities, and overall joy in life. But here's the kicker: you don't need a celebrity-sized bank account to make a difference.

In this book, we're diving into the elite secrets of staying fit and looking youthful. More importantly, I'll show you how to tweak these strategies to fit your budget. You'll discover how to get similar results without breaking the bank.

I get it—you don't have an endless supply of time or money. That's why I'm going to share quick, cost-effective tactics to safeguard your appearance and mental sharpness for years to come.

Chapter 2

Never too Late

You might anticipate that I'd dive straight into some skincare strategies. However, I'm here to say that's just scratching the surface. Sure, it's significant (and reflects broader health), and we'll definitely tackle that topic later in this book.

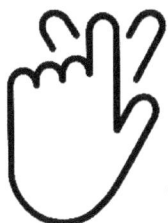

But what's truly crucial is your inner state and your achievements. Your self-perception and outlook on life profoundly influence your appearance, the impression you make on others, and your capabilities. When you feel youthful at heart, it's reflected in your appearance. And if you approach life with vigor and excitement, it makes a world of difference.

The moment we abandon our aspirations and settle for the daily grind is the moment we begin to age. It's having a purpose and zest for life that keeps the inner fire burning, keeping us vibrant and appealing.

So, hold tight to your goals. After all, there's no reason not to…

How our Ambitions and hopes change as we grow

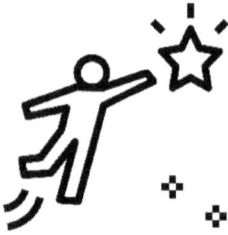

Growing up, many of us had grand aspirations. We imagined ourselves exploring space as astronauts, captivating audiences as rock stars, or perhaps even running our own businesses. However, as we ventured into our twenties, the complexity of turning these dreams into reality became apparent, along with the pressing need for a steady income. Consequently, we settled for more conventional jobs as a temporary solution. Time marches on, and before we know it, we're in our thirties with families or hitting the big four-oh, feeling worn out. It's at this juncture we might concede that those childhood ambitions might remain just that—childhood fantasies. After all, dreams are for the young at heart, aren't they?

The Handy, Strategic Perks That Come with Aging

Many folks reckon that as we age, our dreams slip away, but that's not quite right. Cling to those aspirations, and you'll find they're actually within closer reach as you rack up those birthdays. Why's that? Well, for one, with each passing year, you're piling up experience, which sharpens your know-how in chasing down your goals. Plus, you've had more time to gather some goodies along the way – we're talking cash to back your plans,

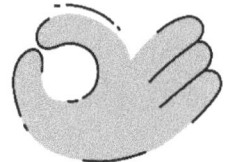

12

a cozy nest egg, a web of contacts, and a resume that packs a punch.

Additionally, you've had ample time to gather valuable resources. This doesn't just mean a healthier bank balance but also a collection of both physical and non-physical assets like real estate, a network of acquaintances, and an impressive resume. If you're enjoying retirement or if the nest is empty with the kids having flown the coop, you've got the gift of time on your hands as well. Mix all these ingredients with a clever understanding of how to make your years' work in your favor, and there's no stopping you from achieving your goals, no matter your age.

Approaches to Accomplishing Remarkable Feats While Maintaining Originality

Countless individuals aspire to become actors, yet often they do not pursue this ambition during their youth. However, with age comes the opportunity to participate in the film industry by applying for roles as an extra or taking on minor characters. As you mature, your availability increases, and interestingly, there is a growing demand for older individuals to fill these niche roles. By accumulating experience and enhancing your resume, you may open unexpected doors in the acting world.

Alternatively, consider leveraging the digital space by launching a YouTube channel. The 'silver surfer' demographic is a substantial segment of the internet population, yet there is a scarcity of targeted content. Creating a fitness channel tailored to those over 50 could potentially garner significant attention and success.

Moreover, with more leisure time at your disposal, writing books and engaging in hobbies become viable options. While becoming an astronaut may be a stretch, participating in a Virgin Galactic flight is within the realm of possibility. If a professional football career is out of reach, coaching or joining a senior team might be a fulfilling alternative.

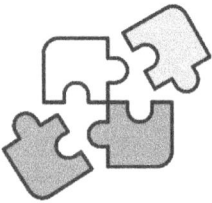

This message is not exclusively for those in their 80s; individuals in their 40s are also well-positioned to take advantage of these insights. Interestingly, the average age of successful startup founders is 40, and the likelihood of starting a prosperous business at 55 is double that of those aged 20-34.

The key is to never surrender to self-imposed limitations. Maintaining health, staving off chronic pain, and keeping your mind agile and sharp will undoubtedly enhance your ability to seize opportunities at any stage of life. A positive mindset and successful endeavors can contribute to a more youthful appearance, and conversely, looking younger can boost your mentality and success. In the following chapter, we will explore strategies to preserve a youthful appearance, supporting your personal and professional goals.

Chapter 3

Strategies for Maintaining a Youthful Appearance Beyond Your Years

Discover secrets to appearing more youthful than your actual years!

Regarding the pursuit of a youthful appearance, the advice you'll encounter generally falls into two distinct groups. One group emphasizes preventative measures to forestall the appearance of aging. Adhering to the adage that prevention surpasses cure, maintaining your skin and sidestepping habits that accelerate aging can sustain your youthful appearance for an extended period.

However, this section is not concerned with preventative strategies. Instead, it delves into the category of recommendations aimed at those who seek to rejuvenate their appearance when signs of aging have already manifested. This section prioritizes practical guidance for enhancing your current appearance because it represents the most direct and effortless route to impact your lifestyle and self-perception positively.

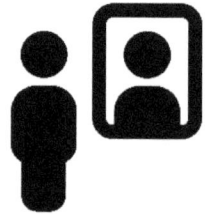

We have considered how adopting a youthful mindset, embracing a vibrant approach to life, and setting youthful expectations can contribute to a sense of, and consequently an appearance of, youthfulness. By implementing these immediate modifications, you can influence how others perceive and interact with you, as well as enhance your own self-image.

Great pointers on maintaining a youthful appearance as the years roll on.

Most people over 20 prefer not to show their true age, and as you edge closer to middle age, each new birthday can feel like a bit of a blow. It's a stark reminder that your dreams of rock stardom are probably behind you, and the chances of dating someone fresh out of high school are dwindling...

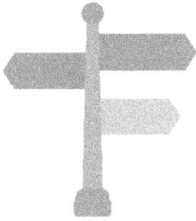

Then there's the not-so-fun part about aging – the changes in your appearance. Witnessing the loss of that once vibrant skin and firm body can feel like a gradual disintegration, and it doesn't help when it feels like society is counting you out. It can be quite disheartening, to say the least.

But here's the silver lining: there are methods to decelerate the aging process and safeguard our skin, so we don't have to broadcast our years to every onlooker. Let's dive into some of these tactics...

Skin Products designed to turn back the clock

Different skincare products have their own methods of action and achieve their goals with mixed results. Keep an eye out for products that boast about having collagen, since the collagen molecules are usually too big to penetrate the pores of your skin.

Similarly, products such as hydrating creams excel at restoring elasticity to our skin, and agents like exfoliating treatments can diminish the visible severity of wrinkles by eliminating lingering dead skin cells from our facial surface. Indeed, should you decide to incorporate a single skincare item to mitigate aging indicators, an exfoliant would be the recommended choice.

Skincare formulations enriched with essential vitamins and minerals can be beneficial. Additionally, many of these products incorporate antioxidants that are applied directly to the skin. It is important to conduct thorough research, including reading consumer feedback and understanding the scientific basis, before selecting a product.

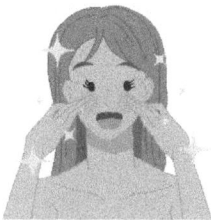

Adopting a strategy to achieve a tanned appearance can be effective in minimizing the visibility of fine lines and wrinkles. This is because a darker skin tone can reduce the contrast between the creases and the surrounding skin, making them less noticeable. However, it is crucial to avoid direct sun exposure, which is a significant factor in accelerating skin aging. Instead, consider using self-tanning hydrators, which are often overlooked. These products gradually tint the skin, offering a healthier and more radiant complexion.

Further exploration of skincare products and their effects will be presented in subsequent sections.

Strategies for Women to Employ Cosmetics for a Youthful Appearance While Embracing Their Present Age

For women using makeup is always an option to cover up

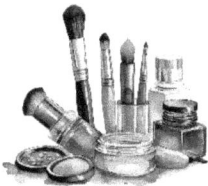

wrinkles and other blemishes. Sure, it's a temporary solution, but it's enough in many cases to make a big difference if you add some foundation to a lined area for example. You should also use this around age spots and other blemishes that might give away your age.

Don't go overboard with foundation though ladies: less is more and it's better to go for a sheer coverage. As you age, matte, powdery foundations can end up building up and clumping in the crags and crevices of your wrinkles and this is not a good look!

Additionally, it's beneficial to minimize the appearance of under-eye bags and creases, which can be achieved using targeted creams that help to rejuvenate these specific areas.

The primary goal for women utilizing makeup to achieve a more youthful look is typically to reintroduce vibrancy to the complexion. As the skin matures, it naturally loses some of its inherent color, leading to a faded or even sickly appearance.

Incorporating color into your makeup routine is effective, yet it's crucial to avoid overly bold contrasts. Opting for vivid eyeshadows or lipsticks can result in an exaggerated, outdated appearance rather than a graceful, age-appropriate one.

The art of using makeup to appear younger lies in the finesse of subtle enhancements. Minor touches, such as a hint of color at the inner eye corners, can have a significant impact.

For a gentle flush, choose a soft peach tone for the cheeks instead of a striking red, ensuring the application is barely perceptible while still making a subconscious impression. Similarly, 'strobing' techniques, which involve applying cream-based highlighters rather than powders, can restore a semblance of youthful glow by accentuating the cheekbones and nose bridge.

When selecting colors for the lips and eyes, aim for shades that offer a gentle contrast to your skin tone. A few shades deeper than your natural complexion can convey a look of elegance and refinement.

Note that dark, matte lip colors may inadvertently thin the appearance of the lips, potentially aging the face. Instead, berry tones and rich, seasonal hues, paired with discreet lip liner and a touch of gloss, can create a fuller, more youthful pout.

Attending a makeup workshop can be highly beneficial. Courses like 'Color Me Beautiful' are designed to equip you with professional makeup application skills tailored to your unique skin tone and features.

Mastering the Art of Charming a Seasoned Romance Enthusiast

Fingers crossed that the tips I just dished out didn't sound like gibberish and you can grasp the potential they have to spruce up your youthfulness vibe. Yet, you may have clocked that a few ladies have tossed this counsel out the window and still manage to dodge the aging bullet.

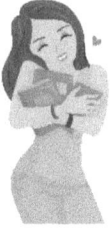

I trust the insights I've shared are clicking with you, and you're beginning to grasp how they could play a role in your quest for a youthful appearance and vibe.

Yet, you've probably clocked that some ladies buck the trend and still manage to look smashing. Take Joanna Lumley, Teri Hatcher, and the entire "Desperate Housewives" crew, or Courtney Cox and Julie Bowen, for example. These women are acing the age-defying look with bolder, more striking makeup choices.

Time has sculpted their faces, sharpening their features to a fine point. Whether through genetics or rigorous fitness and diet routines, they've maintained slender frames, which only accentuates their pronounced cheekbones, deeply set eyes, and slender, more austere lips.

In such instances, the goal is to spotlight those refined features. You might consider going for darker eyebrows, which, contrary to the softer, lighter brows usually associated with youth, can add a dash of drama. opt to make either your eyes or lips pop with a deep, sophisticated hue. And why not dabble in a bit of contouring to bring out those newly defined contours even more? It's like giving your face a high-five with makeup!

Sprucing up your appearance

Alright, folks, perk up your ears! This tidbit is for everyone, but guys, listen up, because it might just hit closer to home. What's the classic hallmark of the distinguished gentleman? That's right, a flourishing garden of nose, ear, and eyebrow hair. And for the ladies reaching a certain vintage, a few sprightly chin whiskers might make an appearance, thanks to our good old friend, hormonal change. But hey, hormones aren't the boss of your grooming routine!

It's all about mindset, really. Letting yourself go is like hanging a sign around your neck that reads, "I'm out of the game and feeling my years." Sure, it's a dead giveaway of your trips around the sun, but it's the psychological effect that really counts. A little snip here and there doesn't just spruce up your look—it's a game-changer. So, wield that trimmer with pride; your mirror (and everyone else) will thank you for it!

Hair Appearance

Our tresses are a defining feature of who we are and how we present ourselves. They're often linked with the essence of youth and vigor, just like a pop of vivid color. Hair sprawls across a significant portion of our skull and peeks out from beneath our attire – making it a loud and clear fashion declaration.

It's no wonder, then, that the emergence of silver strands can revamp our look in a flash – and not always for the better, aging us in the blink of an eye. That's why it's crucial to seek out methods to camouflage those telltale greys. There's a plethora of tactics at our disposal to ensure we maintain a youthful aura and fend off the unwelcome signs of silvering locks.

The go-to strategy for grey camouflage is, of course, hair dye – the more natural, the better. But here's the trick: don't leap to a hue that screams 'unnatural.' Opt for a subtler shade that brightens your natural color while toning down the greys, letting your hair find a happy medium. After all, there's nothing more jarring than spotting an octogenarian with a mane as black as midnight – it screams 'artificial'!

Alternatively, you could hunt for dyes designed to target only the grey hairs. Products like 'Just for Men' might pack some harsh chemicals and get mixed reviews, but they're a step up from blasting your hair with a neon palette.

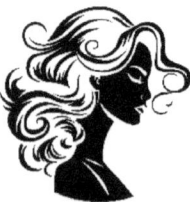

Remember, this is about aging with panache, not spotlighting the greys or trying to rewind your hair's clock back to your teenage days!

For the gents, there's a chic option: owning the grey with a dappled style. A few greys peeking out can look more awkward than a deliberate salt-and-pepper vibe, which, by the way, many find irresistibly dashing. Just look at silver foxes like Matt LeBlanc at 49 and the iconic George Clooney at 56. Ladies, on the flip side, can dip into the silver dye for a 'Mother Nature' vibe, but a snappy short cut might be the key to dodging the 'Earth mother' label.

The Style of your Hair

Switching up your hairdo can play a big part in the age perception game, and it's all about rolling with the years. Ladies, the rule of thumb is: younger gals can rock the Rapunzel look, but as the birthdays pile up, a chic bob might just become your new best friend. For both the gents and the ladies, a trim might be your secret weapon to camouflage thinning locks or those sneaky silver strands. Consider buzzing the sides and letting the top do its thing for a modern twist.

Gentlemen with vanishing manes, it's time to let go. Resist the urge for a flimsy cover-up—nothing screams "denial" like a limp combover. Instead, channel your inner Bruce Willis and own that bald look. It's rugged, it's bold, and hey, it might just add a dash of intimidation to your vibe.

Here's a little style intel for the seasoned gents: while the ladies often chase after a youthful, dewy appearance, you've got a license to flaunt that weathered, grizzled look and still be the guy everyone swoons over. A buzz cut paired with a bit of five o'clock shadow can really nail that seasoned-charm aesthetic.

And let's talk strategy for when your hairline starts to beat a hasty retreat. Cultivating some stubble or a beard is a genius move to shift the spotlight from a barren forehead. It's like a visual declaration that you've still got the vigor to sprout some facial fuzz!

For those fellas not ready to wave the white flag to a receding hairline, consider the 'faux hawk'. Jude Law rocked this style with panache, sporting just a hint of hair strutting down the center of the scalp. It's a subtle nod to the mohawk without going full punk rocker.

Here's a fresh twist on some nifty tricks to shave off a few years from your look in no time...

Lather Up Those Paws - Applying Hand Moisturizer

The state of your hands can be a dead giveaway of your years. Creased mitts can age you faster than a time machine, making you seem older than your driver's license might claim. Keep 'em guessing by slathering on the hand cream like it's going out of style!

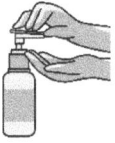

Dress to Impress (Your Age Group).

Forget trying to raid your teenager's closet to turn back the clock. Wearing age-appropriate attire is the real secret to sipping from the fountain of youth. Embrace your current era, don't try to rewind it.

Quench Your Skin's Thirst - Hydrate

If you want to dial back the years instantly, just drink up! Dehydration can turn your skin into a crinkly canvas, showcasing every fine line and vein. Ever wonder why you look like a zombie before your morning coffee? It's because you're parched! And here's a hot tip straight from the fountain of secrets: pop some creatine. Not only will it jazz up your energy levels, but it'll also plump up your skin cells, smoothing out those pesky wrinkles and veins.

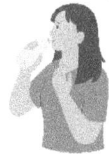

Flash Those Pearly Whites - Teeth

A dazzling smile can be your time-travel device to youth. Ever heard the term 'long in the tooth'? It's no coincidence that teeth are linked with aging. If your champers are more yellow brick road than pearly gates, a trip to the dentist could be your ticket to a younger you. And if you're sporting some gaps, consider dental implants – they might hurt a bit, but they'll iron out those mouth wrinkles in a jiffy.

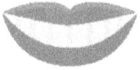

Cosmetic Enhancements (With Caution) - Surgery

Sure, dental work is one kind of nip and tuck that can rewind the years. Veneers are another low-key option to get that Hollywood grin. But when it comes to going under the knife, remember: a little goes a long way. Too much and you might end up looking like a wax figure. So, if you're pondering a face-lift or a Botox bash, think thrice and tread lightly.

Pack on Some Pounds (The Right Way)

Now, I'm not suggesting you become a couch potato, but if you're looking a bit like a human raisin, a few extra pounds could be your saving grace. A little extra cushion can smooth out those lines, and for the gents, it can fend off that fragile look. Just aim for muscle over muffin tops, and you'll be golden.

With these tweaks, you'll be turning heads and sparking "What's their secret?" whispers in no time. Keep it cheeky, keep it classy, and here's to looking fabulous at any age!

Chapter 4

Strategies to Maintain a Youthful Appearance Over Time

Chapter 4 served as an exhaustive manual for immediate youth-enhancing strategies. Should you have implemented the recommendations progressively, it's possible that you've now adopted a more fitting hairstyle, attire, and personal aesthetic. You may have discovered methods to rejuvenate your skin and diminish the visibility of wrinkles and fine lines.

However, the journey doesn't end here. We must now proactively safeguard our appearance against the unyielding advance of time. As previously mentioned, preemptive measures surpass corrective ones. The question remains: How can one effectively halt the aging process in its tracks?

- **Antioxidants**

Antioxidants are substances that counteract the damaging effects of free radicals. Free radicals are unstable molecules that can harm cellular structures by attacking cell membranes, potentially leading to visible signs of aging, such as wrinkles, as well as other skin imperfections like sunspots. Accumulated oxidative damage from free radicals may even contribute to

DNA damage within the cell nucleus, raising the risk of mutations that can lead to cancer.

Antioxidants are abundantly present in various foods and can take numerous forms, including vitamin C found in citrus fruits and omega-6 fatty acids in oily fish. Berries are particularly rich in antioxidants, and incorporating them into one's diet can be conveniently achieved through the consumption of smoothies. These blended beverages can deliver a significant antioxidant dose with little effort and can be cost-effective, as commercial options like those from Innocent may include over twenty berries per bottle, which could be more expensive if purchased and consumed separately.

While smoothies do contain sugar, their benefits often surpass this drawback. It is advisable, however, to limit intake to one smoothie per day. Including these antioxidant-rich drinks in your diet can be a positive step towards better health.

- **Ionized Water for Profound Anti-Aging Effects.**

Several additional strategies exist to enhance the antioxidant advantages of your water. One recommendation is to explore the process of water ionization. Ionized water possesses a greater Oxidation Reduction Potential (ORP), meaning it carries extra electrons which can modify its pH balance, making it less acidic. Consuming water with high acidity levels may contribute to oxidative harm over time, which can lead to premature aging and diminished vitality. To combat this, installing a water ionizer can ensure your water is more conducive to reducing oxidative stress. Many individuals report observing positive changes within a month, and research indicates that such practices could potentially prolong life and diminish age-related signs.

- **Glutathione**

Interested in an advanced tip for combatting aging? It's worth exploring ways to enhance your intake of glutathione through your meals. Glutathione, commonly known as the 'master antioxidant,' is a powerful tripeptide composed of cysteine, glutamic acid, and glycine. Its potency surpasses that of most other antioxidants, playing several vital functions in the body, such as sustaining vitamins C and E (with vitamin E being crucial for skin health), managing the production of hydrogen peroxide, neutralizing lipid peroxide by-products, and aiding in the detoxification process.

So, how can you boost your glutathione levels through diet? It's a bit of a trick question, as glutathione is synthesized internally. However, the encouraging news is that you can enhance its production by consuming more of its precursors. These are the same three amino acids we've discussed: Lcysteine, L-glutamic acid, and glycine. While direct supplementation of cysteine is not advisable due to its potential toxicity, you can derive it from dietary sources such as dairy products, fish, meats, and cheese. Vegetarians can turn to soybeans, spinach, pumpkin, and kale for their intake.

- **Protection**

It is beneficial to minimize instances where your cells might incur damage. This includes limiting sun exposure whenever feasible and refraining from excessive tanning. The sun not only dehydrates our skin but can also inflict additional harm to our cells, accelerating aging and increasing the risk of cancer. Therefore, exercise caution; if you desire a tanned appearance, consider opting for a self-tanning moisturizer as previously recommended. This alternative not only gives you a bronzed look but also helps reflect sunlight, reducing your absorption of it.

Further protective measures include covering up in various ways. For instance, wearing sunglasses is an effective strategy to preserve youthful skin, as they shield the sensitive area around your eyes from damage. This advice echoes the expert recommendations of Aaron Marino, emphasizing the importance of safeguarding your skin to maintain its youthful appearance.

- **Stress**

Acknowledge the profound detrimental effects that stress exerts on your cellular health, neural functions, and the process of aging. Persistent stress ushers in decay, sickness, and accelerated aging. It also fosters inflammation and exacerbates oxidative harm. Stress elevates your heart rate while concurrently hindering both your digestive processes and the efficiency of your immune system. Consequently, if stress is an inescapable aspect of your life, it becomes essential to master stress management techniques. Practicing meditation stands as one of the most efficacious strategies to decelerate the aging process for all the aforementioned reasons.

- **Skin Care and Diet**

Ensure you maintain a healthy skincare routine complemented by a balanced diet as you age. Establish a regimen aimed at shielding your skin from harm and restoring diminished collagen and elastin levels. Regular hydration of your skin is crucial to prevent long-term damage.

The market offers a vast array of skincare products, too numerous to detail here. A useful tip is to seek products that incorporate humectants like hyaluronic acid and vitamin E, which are effective in neutralizing free radicals.

For a dietary addition to lessen the visibility of wrinkles, consider incorporating bone broth into your meals. It is a nutrient-dense option that supports skin elasticity and bone health, rich in collagen, glycine, and minerals such as calcium, phosphorus, and magnesium.

Preparing bone broth involves simmering bones to leach beneficial nutrients into the liquid. Opting for fish bone broth also provides the advantage of iodine content, which can help maintain a healthy thyroid function, potentially aiding in weight management and promoting hair health as you age.

Chapter 5

Maintaining Physical Fitness and Wellness with Advancing Age

Sylvester Stallone has long been an inspiration to me, ever since his groundbreaking role in 'Rocky'. His achievements extend beyond acting; he penned the screenplay and embodied the protagonist without prior acclaim in the film industry. Moreover, his physical transformation for the role galvanized boxers and fitness enthusiasts globally.

Today, Stallone continues to defy expectations. At 66, he appears to be in peak condition, challenging the conventional notions of aging. Despite an age where many enjoy grandparenthood, his physique remains reminiscent of his younger days, offering motivation to those advancing in years.

I'm not suggesting that everyone should emulate Arnold Schwarzenegger or Stallone. That path isn't suitable for the majority. However, I do advocate for an increased focus on exercise as one matures. Regular physical activity not only enhances one's appearance by toning muscles and reducing signs of aging, but it also contributes to a robust appearance, particularly vital for men.

Beyond aesthetics, exercise is instrumental in maintaining cognitive function with age, bolstering overall health, and combating various age-associated conditions like osteoporosis, arthritis, and limited mobility.

So, what's Stallone's secret to maintaining such impressive fitness levels in the face of the typical challenges of aging, including reduced hormones and physical discomfort? Let's explore the probable strategies he employs to maintain his remarkable condition and how you might adopt similar practices.

Conquering the obstacle of maintaining fitness with advancing age.

Hormone

Sylvester Stallone, along with other celebrities, maintains his fitness through the use of growth hormones. While not steroids, growth hormones are a contentious and costly substance, making them impractical for the average person. Nevertheless, there are alternative strategies to enhance your body's innate capabilities for muscle growth and fat reduction, such as various supplements.

One approach is to utilize pro-hormones like testosterone boosters, which stimulate your body to increase testosterone production. This, in turn, can aid in muscle building and fat loss. These supplements are affordable and considered safe, offering a viable option for enhancing physical condition. For younger men, supplements containing ingredients like Tribulus Terrestre's and tong kat ali may not offer tangible benefits. However, older individuals experiencing a natural decline in testosterone may find these supplements significantly advantageous. It should be noted that these are typically recommended for men.

Similarly, boosting growth hormone levels can yield comparable outcomes, benefiting many older men and women. Direct supplementation of growth hormone may not be straightforward, but you can promote its natural production through certain exercises like squats, engaging in high-speed runs, extending sleep duration, and taking hot baths. These practices may be challenging, but they contribute to overall health.

For men seeking peak performance in their later years, hormone therapy with testosterone injections could be a consideration. Nationally, testosterone levels are reportedly decreasing, with the average man having 10% less than a decade ago. This decline is associated with reduced muscle mass, weaker bones, diminished libido, and a higher risk of depression. These issues exacerbate with age, and testosterone injections can potentially revolutionize one's health and well-being.

Joints

As we age, building muscle presents additional challenges, notably increased joint discomfort and the potential for compromised joint integrity due to conditions like arthritis or past injuries. To mitigate joint strain, it's crucial to engage in low-impact exercises, steering clear of activities that could exacerbate joint pain, such as running on hard surfaces. Opting for rowing or cycling can be gentler alternatives. Employing supportive gear can assist in stabilizing your joints during workouts. Prioritizing a thorough warm-up and impeccable exercise technique is now more critical than ever.

Cardiovascular workouts also pose risks to joint health, as high-impact movements can be harsh on them. It's advisable to embrace low-impact cardiovascular activities, such as brisk walking, swimming, or using a recumbent bicycle to maintain joint health while staying active.

Energy

Training in advanced years can be challenging, even for those in peak physical condition, as fatigue and energy depletion may become more pronounced during exercise. Nonetheless, enhancing one's energy levels is possible through improved nutritional strategies, such as incorporating energy-boosting supplements like energy beverages and creatine, or by prioritizing adequate rest and extended sleep.

Should muscle soreness persist following a workout, it's prudent to moderate the intensity of subsequent exercise sessions, ensuring ample rest and a diet rich in protein before focusing on the same muscle groups once more.

Furthermore, it's worth emphasizing the benefits of low-impact activities such as walking, swimming, or utilizing a recumbent bicycle. These exercises serve as excellent alternatives for maintaining an active lifestyle, particularly when more vigorous training methods become less feasible with age.

Maintaining Movement, Vitality, and Wellness Throughout the Lifespan

Consider embracing yoga or even gymnastics as part of your routine. Shortly, you'll discover the significance of physical activity for cognitive health, as well as its vital role in maintaining bodily function. A primary cause of joint issues in later years is the prolonged periods of inactivity, particularly sitting, which is contrary to the body's natural design, coupled with insufficient movement.

This sedentary lifestyle leads to increased joint stiffness, tendon shortening and lengthening, and muscle atrophy. These changes can result in uneven stress on joints and, over time, contribute to the reduced mobility often associated with aging.

The principle is straightforward: maintain an active lifestyle to preserve your mobility. If you've noticed a decrease in your mobility, it's essential to gradually reintroduce movement into your life.

Moreover, for those who are young and in good health, incorporating High-Intensity Interval Training (HIIT) into your fitness regimen is advisable. HIIT consists of alternating between high-intensity exercise bursts and slower recovery periods. This not only fortifies your heart and enhances your VO2 max, potentially lowering the risk of heart disease—the leading cause of death in the Western world—but also boosts the quantity and efficiency of your mitochondria. These cellular 'power plants' are responsible for converting glucose into ATP, the energy currency of the cell.

The abundance of mitochondria in children is one reason they have seemingly endless energy compared to adults. Engaging in HIIT can increase your mitochondrial count and enhance the efficiency of your energy metabolism, thereby reducing oxidative stress.

To learn more about HIIT, consider researching it online. Pairing HIIT with stretching, mobility exercises (as outlined in "Becoming a Supple Leopard"), and incorporating long walks, fresh air, and weight training can greatly enhance your physical strength and vitality. This holistic approach to fitness not only improves your appearance and energy levels but also helps in preventing a wide array of health issues

Chapter 6

Maintain cognitive acuity and mental agility as you mature to prevent intellectual property infringement.

Growing older often brings a host of unwelcome changes, and while we may primarily concern ourselves with the physical decline, the deterioration of cognitive abilities can be even more distressing. The gradual onset of forgetfulness and a noticeable deceleration in our cognitive processes can lead to significant distress and a sense of isolation, even in the absence of specific illnesses like dementia.

However, this decline in mental acuity is not an inescapable fate. With dedication and effort, it is possible to fortify the mind and maintain its youthfulness, akin to exercising a muscle. In this discussion, we will explore strategies to enhance mental sharpness and mitigate the cognitive impairments often associated with aging.

Exercise

Engaging in physical activity is a crucial strategy for maintaining strength and wellness in your body during the aging process, a fact we have previously established. However, the advantages of exercise extend beyond the apparent physical benefits. Significantly, it serves to fortify cognitive function. For those experiencing challenges with short-term memory due to aging, it's noteworthy that enhancing memory is a primary benefit of initiating an exercise program, particularly one with a focus on cardiovascular workouts. Given our prior exploration of optimal training methods for the aging population, this additional incentive underscores the importance of adhering to the recommended exercise plan.

Use

The adage 'exercise it or risk losing it' certainly holds true in this context. Actively engaging our minds through imaginative exercises is among the most effective strategies to prevent cognitive decline. Activities that require strategic planning and the manipulation of numbers are particularly beneficial. For instance, strategic games like chess or certain video games are excellent choices. However, any intellectual activity, including occasional reading, can be advantageous.

By participating in these activities, you are enhancing what's known as 'working memory,' which is essential for 'fluid intelligence.' Fluid intelligence is the adaptive form of intelligence that tends to diminish with age.

Diet

A proper nutritional regimen is essential for maintaining cognitive health and staving off various neurodegenerative conditions or general cognitive decline. Omega-3 fatty acids are particularly beneficial; these can be sourced from seafood and dietary supplements. Omega-3s enhance the fluidity of cell membranes, fostering better neuronal communication, and they also counteract inflammation, which can harm the brain. Essential nutrients like vitamin B9 (folic acid), found in fruits and vegetables, and amino acids, derived from meats or supplements, are crucial for synthesizing vital neurotransmitters that support memory and cognitive functions.

However, the list of dietary components that positively influence brain health is extensive. Magnesium contributes to relaxation and the brain's ability to adapt and change, while lutein has been linked to memory preservation and ocular health in later life. Additionally, choline, obtained from eggs, is a precursor to acetylcholine, a neurotransmitter that modulates brain activity. The inventory of brain-supporting nutrients is indeed exhaustive.

A well-balanced diet is crucial for preserving mental acuity and warding off a range of neurodegenerative diseases or general declines in mental function. Particularly advantageous are omega-3 fatty acids, which are obtainable through fish and nutritional supplements. These acids improve the pliability of cellular membranes, which enhances communication between neurons, and they also mitigate inflammation that can damage the brain. Vitamins such as B9 (folic acid), present in produce, along with amino acids from proteins or supplements, are vital for the production of important neurotransmitters that bolster memory and cognitive capabilities.

Yet, the array of nutritional elements that have a positive impact on brain health is comprehensive. Magnesium plays a role in relaxation and the brain's capacity for neuroplasticity, while lutein is associated with the retention of memory and eye health in the aging process. Furthermore, choline, sourced from eggs, serves as a building block for acetylcholine, a neurotransmitter that regulates cerebral activity. The list of nutrients that support brain function is indeed extensive.

Lifestyle

Your lifestyle choices can significantly influence your mental health. Adequate sleep and exposure to fresh air play a vital role in brain health, while excessive alcohol consumption can be detrimental. Adopting habits that promote brain health will enhance the benefits of a nutritious diet and other positive changes. It's important to recognize that even minor damage accumulated over time can lead to serious health issues.

Substances like alcohol and tobacco are particularly harmful. Not only do they accelerate physical aging, leading to symptoms such as discolored teeth and early wrinkles, but they also have the potential to destroy brain cells. Similarly, insufficient sleep and high stress levels can cause considerable harm to both your physical and mental well-being, hastening cell death and compromising your immune system.

An often-neglected aspect of brain health is the risk of physical injury. Research shows a clear link between traumatic brain injuries and the development of neurological conditions like Parkinson's disease and dementia. Athletes in high-impact sports frequently suffer from brain injuries that may affect their long-term health. Moreover, everyday incidents such as falls or vehicle accidents can cause subtle brain damage that might go unnoticed. Many people may be living with minor brain injuries without realizing it.

Therefore, it is crucial to protect your brain by wearing helmets, avoiding high-impact sports that can cause concussions, and generally taking care of your brain's well-being. Remember, your brain is both incredibly vital and remarkably delicate.

The Essential Method for Maintaining a Youthful and Robust Mind during Advanced Years

Implementing various changes can contribute to maintaining robust cognitive functions as you grow older. However, these elements are not the most crucial for brain health. The primary factor is continuous learning and exposure to novel experiences. To grasp this concept, one must understand the brain's fundamental purpose. Essentially, the brain is a sophisticated learning apparatus, designed through evolution to enable us to adapt and adjust our behavior to our environment. It is this ability to learn and adapt that has been essential for human survival.

This capability is made possible by what is known as 'neuroplasticity,' which is the brain's capacity to form new neural connections and even generate new neurons in response to stimuli.

Engaging with new and stimulating activities triggers the release of neurotransmitters such as dopamine and norepinephrine, which sharpen our focus and attention. Concurrently, levels of BDNF (brain-derived neurotrophic factor) and nerve growth factor rise, both critical for neuroplasticity and the formation of new neural pathways.

However, if we cease to challenge our brains with fresh experiences, we hinder the production of these vital hormones and neurotransmitters, leading to a decline in their release over time. This decline can result in the brain's growth halting and its gradual deterioration.

The adage that 'you can't teach an old dog new tricks' stems from the fact that as we age, we often expose ourselves to fewer novel challenges.

A child's brain exhibits remarkable plasticity as it acquires fundamental skills such as walking, speaking, and playing. Similarly, young adults retain a high degree of plasticity as they learn to navigate driving, new job roles, and more.

However, the brain's learning pace can decelerate when one has been in the same role for many years, with fewer opportunities for learning. This slowdown is exacerbated if physical mobility is impaired due to joint damage or conditions like arthritis. Physical movement is a potent brain stimulus, and its absence, coupled with reduced exploration and social interaction, can lead to depression, irritability, memory issues, and potentially dementia.

Therefore, it is imperative to persist in acquiring new knowledge, mastering languages, developing skills, and coding languages, as well as to continue socializing and exploring new environments. Pursuing goals is also vital. It's important to remember that it's never too late to achieve what you've always aspired to be.

Chapter 7

Is it Possible that the Individual Destined for Immortality is Already Among Us?

Are you aware of a jellyfish species with biological immortality? This organism, known as Turritopsis dohrnii, can theoretically evade death indefinitely, barring predation or disease. Its remarkable capability stems from its ability to revert to its juvenile polyp stage, essentially resetting its life cycle and regenerating its cells, akin to a rejuvenation process reminiscent of the fictional Dr. Who.

While the implications of this phenomenon for human longevity are speculative, it underscores a fascinating possibility. As we continue to explore the mechanisms of aging and regeneration, some experts propose that the first human capable of eternal life may already be among us. The feasibility and mechanisms behind this potentiality remain subjects of scientific inquiry and debate.

Why it Might be Possible

As individuals gain more knowledge about maintaining wellness, combating diseases, and enhancing our nutrition and overall lifestyles, the human lifespan continues to extend. With reductions in smoking, enhancements in dietary habits, access to purer water, and advancements in medical treatments, we are witnessing lifespans that surpass those from a century ago. The longest confirmed lifespan to date reached an extraordinary 122 years and 164 days. Given the potential for this record to be surpassed, it is plausible to consider that individuals born in the current era may achieve lifespans of 130 to 140 years, potentially passing away around the year 2153. By that time, it is anticipated that technology will have evolved to a state far beyond our current comprehension. Technological progress, as suggested by Moore's Law, which posits that technological growth is exponential, not linear, is expected to make even more significant strides in the upcoming century than it has in the past.

Some Popular Life Extension Techniques

In the current era, it is anticipated that the advent of new medical treatments and technological advancements could significantly enhance our way of living. There is a growing body of evidence pointing towards this possibility, with numerous potential breakthroughs on the horizon. For example, research conducted by the Institute of Regenerative Medicine in Pittsburgh has shown a remarkable 200% increase in the lifespan of mice following stem cell injections from younger specimens. Given the success of these experiments in rodents, it seems plausible that human trials could be on the horizon, potentially within the next century or sooner.

Furthermore, innovative approaches to longevity, such as gene doping to bolster mitochondrial resilience and efficiency, have been explored. These powerhouses of the cell are crucial for energy production and safeguarding against oxidative stress. Projections indicate that such interventions could not only add up to 30% to our lifespan but also fortify us against diseases like cancer and reduce susceptibility to injuries such as burns.

Another promising area of research involves telomeres, the protective caps at the ends of our chromosomes. These structures shield our genetic material during cell division, but they shorten over time, leading to the aging process once they are depleted. Techniques aimed at restoring telomere length could potentially offer a method to delay aging and extend human life.

Imagine this...

Let us consider the possibility that within the next 140 years, the adoption and efficacy of various life-extending techniques are established. Theoretically, this could enable your descendants to increase their lifespans by 300%, potentially living up to 420 years. They would likely experience fewer health issues, and if they did fall ill, they would benefit from advanced medical interventions.

Fast forward to the year 2432, where it is conceivable that even more sophisticated technologies could emerge, offering further lifespan enhancements or potentially eternal life. However, this optimistic scenario is not guaranteed; human self-destruction through nuclear conflict or a decline in health due to sedentary lifestyles and excessive dependence on technology are real risks that could curtail such advancements.

Despite the uncertainty, the notion that the first being capable of immortality might already exist is quite extraordinary, and while improbable, it is not entirely outside the realm of possibility that this being could be you.

In the interim, it is imperative to prioritize your health and vitality. Adhering to the guidance provided in this text is crucial. Embrace it and make it a cornerstone of your life. It may indeed be the key to unlocking an unprecedentedly long existence.

ABOUT AUTHOR

Maya Genn is An Author and expert in health, skincare and fitness, committed to guiding people achieving their wellness aspirations and leading energetic, fulfilling lives. Her expertise is rooted in beauty, science and Holistic wellness, which she uses to enrich her writing, steering her audience toward peak health, vigor and radiant skin.

Maya's writing is driven by a desire to inspire positive transformations, helping readers cultivate healthy habits, navigate skincare routines, and make informed choices that support their overall well-being. Whether demystifying the latest skincare trends or delving into the science of nutrition, Maya's engaging voice and expertise shine through, offering readers valuable guidance on their journey to optimal health and radiant skin.

Through her articles, books, and online platforms, Maya continues to share her passion for health and skincare, empowering readers worldwide to embrace self-care, confidence, and natural beauty from the inside out.

www.ingramcontent.com/pod-product-compliance
Lightning Source LLC
Chambersburg PA
CBHW052123030426

42335CB00025B/3086